Author's Note:

Please consult your physician before beginning this or any other diet program. Our bodies are all different. Any decision affecting your health is personal and should be made only after talking with your doctor or other health professional.

There is no way that I can guarantee that weight loss success will come for everyone who reads this book. I <u>can</u> guarantee that the people most likely to be successful are those who dive into the program with enthusiasm. I strongly urge you to keep learning as much as you can about the newest discoveries about diet and nutrition, so you can make conscious, well-informed choices about your health.

If you are diabetic your doctor may decide that this diet contains too many carbohydrates for you. Although the diet has no white sugar or flour, there is more fruit, whole grains and bread than some diabetic specialists recommend. If you wish to use the Easy-Does-It Diet's simplicity and convenience, work with your doctor to fine-tune the program to your own dietary needs. This is healthy advice for anyone with chronic health problems related to their diet or lifestyle.

Table of Contents

Easy-Does-It

_____

Why Do You Need This Book?

I love reading the many emails I receive from readers of the *How to Think Thin Newsletter* and my previous book *Weight Loss: How to Keep Your Commitment*. This email I received from Darcy said it so well for so many:

> Hi Jonni,
>
> I'm a 32 yr old single mom and I just got accepted to University and am starting this fall. I have gained about 50+ lbs in the past year and a half and I'm so frustrated… I don't have a lot of money … so what I'm asking is off the cuff do you have any advice?? I really don't want to start my new life FAT!!!
>
> Please help,
> Darcy

Readers like Darcy have made it clear to me that excess weight is only *one* problem that we have to deal with. We each have many things to worry about in addition to our weight – after all, the rest of life isn't going to stop and wait for us while we find a good diet and figure out how to use it.

For most people the ideal weight loss plan would be both simple *and* affordable. Difficult-to-understand diet programs with too many choices and expensive ingredients just add to our stress, and often cause us to give up on a diet before we even get started.

Companies like Jenny Craig®, L A Weight Loss® and NutriSystem® have recognized the need for an easy, no-fuss diet program, and they offer a 'simple' solution: Buy their pre-made meals, pop them in your freezer, and follow their daily menu plans. The meals are formulated to give you a specific daily calorie count that will help most people lose their unwanted pounds – at least for a while.

These programs are a great idea – *but they're expensive*. Most people find it difficult to take money from their family's monthly food budget to spend up to $300 for meals that no one else can eat.

An alternative to the fancy packaged diets can be found at the local supermarket in the freezer case. Brands like Healthy Choice®, Weight-Watchers®, and Stouffer's Lean Cuisine® are very popular, especially with people who have access to a microwave oven at lunchtime. The meals are reasonably tasty, very convenient, and contain fewer calories and fat than a sandwich or meal from your local lunch counter.

However, if you add up the cost of these frozen meals, you'll see you're still spending a lot of money for the convenience, and many of these diet meals leave you hungry.

Think about it – what these companies are really charging you for is the fixed portions. They put less on your plate than you would normally serve yourself. They give you the will-power by making your choices for you, but it lets them charge you more money for less food!

The Easy-Does-It Alternative

The Easy-Does-It Diet uses the simplicity of the prepared diet plans with a simple twist – *you* make the meals yourself, so *you* control the quality, *you* control the taste, and the delicious meals you prepare yourself cost about **1/3rd** as much as the manufactured low-fat meals from the supermarket – and **1/5th** the cost of the packaged diets from the big weight loss companies!

What this means is that you can have all the convenience and benefits of the high-priced prepared meal plans, but at a huge savings. I was excited to discover that the healthiest food are actually some of the least expensive foods to buy, so this plan actually allows you spend less money than you would when you're *not* dieting. The cost savings, along with the health benefits, add up to a fantastic way to feed your whole family.

But the lower cost is not the only benefit of this program.

Many people I've spoken to have loved the weight loss results they experience while using the regulated programs like Jenny Craig® or Weight-Watchers®. But, sooner or later, they run out of money for the special food – or they find they can't afford the time to go to the meetings. When they go off the program they start gaining weight again because they go back to eating like they did in the past.

The Easy-Does-It Diet is a *do-it-yourself* program, so you'll be building new, healthy habits as you prepare your meals. The plan is so convenient, and so inexpensive, that you'll have fewer excuses for giving up. And you'll be learning how to make healthy choices on your own. You can give yourself and your family a lifetime of good health.

This is not a low-calorie, quick weight loss plan. It's been proven for years that reducing the calories too much *will* help you lose weight temporarily – but it *also* changes your metabolic rate so that you regain weight quickly when the diet is over. Most people gain more weight than they lost, and end up heavier than they were when they started. I didn't want to call this *The Yo-Yo Diet Book*, so you won't be counting calories.

What you will be doing is what almost all nutritional experts recommend: Eat a healthy diet filled with fresh salads, steamed vegetables and beans and eat in moderation. You'll not only lose your weight safely, but you won't be putting yourself on that weight loss-and-gain roller coaster. If you're already on that ride, this diet will let you get off, so you can regain your health.

To follow the plan you'll need to buy some plastic containers in three or four different sizes, and you'll need to have access to a microwave. You'll also need a few hours every month when you'll create your own delicious pre-packaged diet meals. After that, it's all Easy-Does-It!

I first created the Easy-Does-It Diet for myself. I work at a full-time, high-stress job as a customer service representative at the largest health insurance company in the state. And I have a home-based business that requires at least 20 more hours a week, writing my *How to Think Thin Newsletter* and responding to my reader's questions and concerns. Plus, I like to read a good book as often as possible, I have two cats that demand some attention occasionally, and I have a deck crammed with growing plants. Add a few social activities and visiting with friends and family, and who has time to worry about what to eat?

In order to have time for all these activities, I needed to simplify my life as much as possible. Although my particular interests and problems are different from yours, you will have just as many things going on in your life as I do – probably more.

Because I love to read, and I've always been interested in health issues, I've read a whole bookshelf full of books on diets and nutrition. The books were written over a long period of time – I've read works by authors who were famous at the beginning of the last century, along with book just hot off the press. And I've read books that run the gamut of weight loss theory – including Norman Walker's juicing and fasting ideas, Dr Atkins' high-fat, low-carb plan, and Drs Fuhrman and Ornish, who encourage low-fat meals based on plant foods.

Now, you know that reading a large number of diet books doesn't make anyone an expert, but I have found some interesting things during my armchair research. Although fads come and go in the health field, just like anything else, there are constants that you'll find in almost every book on nutrition and weight loss. You might be surprised to discover that "calories", and the need for fewer of them, is not considered important by all authors. In fact, it has been known for some time that eating a very low calorie diet will lower your resting metabolism – which causes you to regain your excess weight – and more! – as soon as you go back to eating normally. In fact, the diet book that has taken Europe by storm, *Eat Yourself Slim* by Michel Montignac, suggests that the 'calorie theory' is false.

If you've spent any length of time battling your weight, you know that a low-calorie diet that simply reduces the amount of food you eat, without changing the *way* you eat, will only work for a short time. Sooner or later you'll regain the weight and become one of the millions of people on the yo-yo diet.

One thing *all* the diet books have said is that we need healthy, wholesome, nutritious food, *in moderation* – along with regular exercise – to build a thin, healthy body that will stay active and energetic for many years. The foods that help build that wonderfully healthy body are the fresh salad greens, the amazing variety of steamed vegetables, and beans. Yes, the lowly bean has been called the weight loss miracle by many experts, such as Dr. Joel Fuhrman, author of *Eat to Live*. And even the low-carb proponents encourage us to eat lots of healthy raw and steamed vegetables.

I've put together a plan that uses the ideas that all the diet books hold in common. Putting those themes into a simple, easy to follow eating plan took several years of experimentation and creativity, and resulted in the program I now personally follow. I used it in the beginning because I had an extra 30 pounds to get rid of. Once I reached a healthy weight, I still continued to use this program. It's the reason why I have not regained the 30 pounds I lost like I always did in the past.

While putting the plan together, I felt that there were some criteria that had to be met in order for the plan to fit my concept of the 'ideal' diet:

1. It has to be easy. Otherwise, I would need to change the title of the book to *The Complicated Diet That Requires a Lot of Reading and Math.*

2. It has to contain all foods that people normally eat, with a few simple exceptions. And since we all have different traditions, the diet needs to be flexible so that you can tailor it to your own tastes and dietary needs.

3. There has to be plenty of food. Feeling deprived is not conducive to good health, mentally or physically. While moderation is important, (and we sometimes need to tell ourselves "no"), we should always know that we're getting enough food to satisfy our needs.

4. It has to be nutritious. That means that all food groups are represented, with nothing left out. The food needs to contain more vitamins, minerals and micronutrients than the 'normal' American diet contains, and it needs to have far more fiber. These nutrients and fiber will help to wash the fat out of your body, and they help strengthen your immune system.

5. It has to be self-regulating. It needs to be easy to know how to change the diet in order to fit with your own personal needs. Some people work harder than others, and need more food. Some people need less.

6. It has to be easy. Oh, did I say that already?

What Do You Eat?

Here is the basic plan, as I personally follow it:

Breakfast:

- Fruit and one slice of whole grain bread

- Or fruit and oatmeal with raisins and soy or skim milk
- Or one fruit smoothie made with frozen fruit and soy milk, with a small amount of honey

Lunch:

- Large salad and one cup bean soup, with one slice whole grain bread, plus fruit
- Or large whole meal salad with one slice whole grain bread, plus fruit
- Or Large salad with one Easy-Does-It frozen meal with beans, plus fruit

Dinner:

- Large salad with one Easy-Does-It frozen meal with chicken or meat, plus fruit

Snacks:

- Fruit or fruit smoothie made with skim or soy milk and small amount of honey.
- Or raw vegetables, such as carrots, celery and broccoli

Each lunch and dinner should begin with a very large salad, and each day you will eat at least one cup of beans or bean soup. The beans can be added to your whole-meal salad, eaten as one of the delicious soups you'll be placing in single-serving containers and placing in your freezer, or in an Easy-Does-It frozen entrées. Because most of us add honey to our smoothies, you should eat only one smoothie a day – make it your special treat to look forward to.

This diet emphasizes the kinds of food that many experts believe will help you lose weight. It does not emphasize the kinds of foods that you should avoid, but it's important to know what the diet is leaving out.

- **Sugar** and all refined starchy foods – which means all **white flour, white rice,** and processed foods made with these ingredients

That's a pretty short list, but it's an important one. The World Health Association has recently released a report that shows that obesity is one of the top 10 causes of preventable disease and death, world-wide. Their recommendation is to eat much more fruits and vegetables than most people do now, and to eat far less sugar and refined grains.

These products, (I hate to call them 'food'), have been stripped of all nutritional value and go straight to your hips. They also add to your potential of getting heart disease, diabetes and cancer. There are no known benefits to these products, and many reasons to avoid them. They are not included in this diet.

What if This is Too Much food?

The whole grain bread is the first thing to leave out if you can't eat this much food or if you don't lose weight as fast as you'd like to. You can add the bread back into your diet once you've reached your ideal weight. Many experts don't recommend the low-carb diets because the high amounts of protein can damage your kidneys and the high fat can lead to heart disease and some kinds of cancer. But Dr. Atkins and other low-carb proponents do have one thing right – the fastest, cheapest way to get fat is to lay on the carbohydrates, especially the refined starches and sugars that fill most processed foods.

If you doubt that carbohydrates will make you fat, just buy a whole chicken from the supermarket. Cut it up and notice the huge globs of fat that hang on every piece of the bird – even the heart and liver. If you want your own innards to look like that, you can load up on wheat and corn products, like the chicken was forced to do.

However, *reasonable* amounts of *unrefined* whole grains and potatoes give you lots of nutrients besides plain old calories, and may be included in moderation.

You may also need to replace some of the fruit snacks with cut-up raw vegetables if you aren't losing as much weight as you'd like. Just be sure to eat *some* fruit every day.

Be sure to eat as much salad and steamed vegetables as you can, because these foods will help you lose weight and will help you feel full so that your body doesn't go into survival mode, as it does with so many quick-weight loss diets. Long term health should be your goal.

If quick weight loss is really your aim, I strongly suggest that you make a point of drinking lots of fresh water, and cut back or eliminate the caffeine. Coffee and cola drinks can actually dehydrate you, and your cells will fight back by trying to hold on to the water that's left. This prevents your cells from completely flushing toxins out of your system, and can add an extra 5 to ten pounds to your weight.

Drinking lots of water lets the cells clean themselves out, and the extra water flushes out of your system. It doesn't just help you look better — it also keeps you healthy.

What if This Isn't Enough Food?

If you lose too much weight or feel hungry after your meal, eat a cup of bean soup *and* an Easy-Does-It frozen meal along with a very large salad. Some active teenagers and adults who have very physical jobs may want two frozen meals for dinner. You will know if you're getting enough by the way you feel after your meal, and by the numbers on your bathroom scale. You won't be counting calories, and you won't be keeping a diet journal. But you can tell if you're eating too much simply by noticing if you lose weight or not.

If you feel hungry, but you don't want to change the diet too much because you like the amount of weight you're losing, eat a larger salad and make it as exciting as you can. You can also throw in an extra container of steamed vegetables. You can't eat too many steamed vegetables, unless you insist on eating nothing but potatoes. There is no excuse for not having enough to eat on the Easy-Does-It Diet.

What's an Easy-Does-It Frozen Meal?

Actually, you can use just about any recipe that you love and build an Easy-Does-It frozen meal. The 'magic' is in the proportions — you will use the same size container for all your meals and fill three quarters of your container with vegetables. You won't be doing any chopping, washing, cutting, peeling or picking of these vegetables, unless you want to – I always use two 16 oz packages (or equivalent) of whatever cut-and-mixed frozen vegetables I find on sale on my shopping day to fill 6 Easy-Does-It frozen meals. I've included a number of recipes for Easy-Does-It frozen meals so that you can get into the hang of building your own inexpensive and healthy entrées. Once you see how easy it is to use these meals you'll soon be adapting your own recipes. Naturally, you'll want to use low-fat cooking methods for your own recipes.

As long as you always fill ¾ of the container with vegetables, use approximately 3 oz. or less of any meat or chicken, and limit your grain (whole grain rice, bulgur, whole grain noodles, potatoes, etc.) to ½ cup, you'll have a healthy meal when eaten with a large salad. Add fruit for desert. You'll be eating what you love, in healthy quantities, and you should never feel picked on or deprived.

Your bean soups and bean entrées are just as important as your frozen meals with meat – even more important, really. Actually, Americans don't eat anywhere near enough beans in order to stay healthy – but this diet will change all that. Beans help you lose weight, and some beans have been found to have anti-cancer properties. And they're cheap. What more could we ask for? I have included a number of excellent recipes for bean soups and entrées, all using fast-cooking beans or canned beans, so you won't be slaving over a hot stove on your weekend. (Or we'd have to call this *The Hard Work Diet*.)

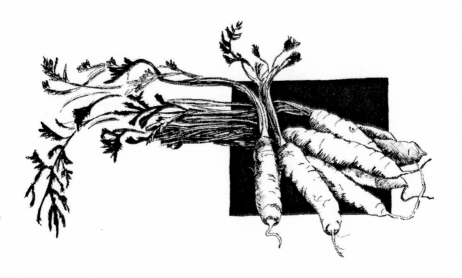

Why Make Your Own?

If you work in an office that offers a microwave oven in the break-room, you're probably familiar with the "healthy" frozen meals offered by **Healthy Choice®**, **Weight-Watchers®**, **Stouffer's Lean Cuisine®**, and other companies.

You may already buy these products because you get an easy low-cal lunch that can be easily eaten at your desk or in the lunch room. They also cost less than meals at the local restaurant.

So why make your own? There are actually several very good reasons:

- You control the quality.

- You control the taste.

- You control the portion sizes.

- You save a lot of money.

What's in Their Frozen meals?

I checked the ingredients list for Stouffer's Lean Cuisine® Honey Roasted Pork with Roasted Gold Potatoes. Here's what's in this product:

> Roasted potatoes, water, seasoned cooked pork product (pork, water, coating), dehydrated honey (sugar, honey), maltodextrin, partially hydrogenated cottonseed and soybean oil, modified food starch, dehydrated garlic, salt, fructose, corn syrup solids, dehydrated flavor (nonfat dry milk, gum Arabic), wheat soybeans, why protein concentrate, salt, flavor (canola oil, natural flavors), onion juice, potassium chloride, dextrose, honey flavor (honey, ethyl alcohol, water, propylene glycol, flavor), lemon juice powder (maltodextrin, lemon juice concentrate, lemon oil, natural flavorings), carrots, red peppers, honey, soy sauce (water, wheat, soybeans, salt, lactic acid), modified cornstarch, butter, roasted garlic concentrate (garlic, salt, natural flavoring, sesame oil, canola oil and citric acid), onions, bleached enriched wheat flour (wheat flour, niacin, iron, thiamin mononitrate, riboflavin, folic acid), garlic puree, salt, flavoring (maltodextrin, yeast extract, cultured whey, flavor, and salt), spices, potassium chloride, caramel coloring, erythorbic acid, sugar, carrageenan with dextrose.

Wow...You probably wouldn't cook a meal that contained "seasoned cooked pork product" or "erythorbic acid" for your family. (What is erythorbic acid, anyway?)

Your Easy-Does-It Frozen Meal

Here's the list, using the national labeling standard that requires the major ingredients to be listed first:

- **Red potatoes**
- **Broccoli**
- **pork**
- **honey**
- **soy sauce**
- **prepared mustard.**

That sounds a little more appetizing, doesn't it?

You're in Control

Let's face it – to mass-produce a frozen meal that is profitable, the manufacturer needs to keep a close eye on the bottom line. The portions in the average "healthy" frozen lunch may be chosen more to save the company money than to reduce the calories. You finish your meal feeling hungry, and find yourself poking quarters in the candy machine during your next break.

By using containers with more room you can come close to doubling the quantity and nutrition of your meals simply by adding a good-sized portion of vegetables. You won't get up from the table hungry.

Better Taste

Mass-produced frozen meals need to appeal to millions of people – and we all have different tastes. That's probably why most of the frozen meals are so bland.

Your own meals will be custom-made to appeal only to you and the others in your family who will eat them. That means you can add herbs, spices and other flavors to make meals that you will truly enjoy.

The meals you create might not appeal to the people down the street, or across the country, but they'll be perfect for you and your family!

Less Fat

Yes, less fat in the diet will definitely help you lose weight. You'll also want to restrict the fat in your diet because excess fat has been associated with an increased risk of both heart disease and cancer.

According to Dr. Christiane Northrup, author of *Women's Bodies, Women's Wisdom: Crating Physical and Emotional Health and Healing*, scientists have know since 1977 that the countries where people eat the most animal fat are also the countries that have the highest breast cancer rate. Other researchers have connected dietary fat with heart disease and other types of cancers, especially those that respond to hormones, like prostate cancer.

This is one of the biggest reasons why dietary experts such as Dr. Dean Ornish recommend a diet that relies exclusively on plants. However, I recognize that any change in your diet needs to fit in with your family's needs and expectations, as well as your own – and many people find it very difficult to give up the recipes and foods that they're used to and go completely vegetarian.

Therefore, this diet includes small portions of chicken and meat, but you'll also find non-meat options. You may wish to gradually reduce the meals that include meat, or you may choose to continue to keep meat in your diet as a special treat. Just remember to use the meat or chicken as the Chinese do – as flavoring, instead of the main part of the meal.

More Fiber

One automatic benefit of a diet high in green salads, steamed vegetables, beans and whole grains is *fiber*. Recent research has found that even small increases in daily fiber intake can reduce cholesterol levels and reduce the risk of heart disease.

Dr. Joel Fuhrman, author of *Eat to Live,* is very excited about the benefits of fiber. He says that although the TV commercials for Metamucil make us think of fiber as something gritty and unpleasant tasting, this really isn't what dietary fiber is all about. By including foods that are unprocessed, without the natural fiber removed, we can eliminate such health problems as hemorrhoids, constipation, varicose veins and diabetes – and reduce the chances of getting colon cancer, a major killer in America. Most of us don't get enough fiber because we eat too many processed foods and too few fruits, vegetables, beans and whole grains.

This is one area where our **Easy-Does-It Diet** outshines the mass-produced weight loss meals. The large companies are concerned with low calories and high profits. They need to keep their meals as "normal" as possible for the American public so they rely on low-fiber noodles and white rice, which are inexpensive fillers, but very low in dietary fiber and nutrition. The **Easy-Does-It Diet** gives you the fiber that your body needs.

More Nutrition

You can see that this diet is not *just* about losing weight — although that is a very nice result of following this plan. The simplicity and convenience of the plan makes it easy to include far more nutrition than most Americans are used to — and your body will notice the positive change. You may discover that you have more energy, which will allow you to get out and exercise more — which will help improve your metabolism so you'll lose weight even faster. You may find your moods are more stable, that you feel 'down' less often. Perhaps you'll be able to withstand stressful situations more easily. A healthy diet can have wonderful effects on all aspects of life.

Less Money

On a recent Saturday afternoon I cooked an entire freezer-full of healthy Easy-Does-It frozen meals. Here's what they cost, along with the cost of similar commercial meals:

Healthy Choice® Sweet and Sour Chicken $2.99
Easy-Does-It Sweet and Sour Chicken   **$1.21**

Healthy Choice® Country Herb Chicken	$2.99
Easy-Does-It Country Herb Chicken	**$1.11**
Stouffer's Lean Cuisine® Chicken & Vegetables	$3.49
Easy-Does-It Chicken & Vegetables	**$1.02**
Stouffer's Lean Cuisine® Honey Roasted Pork	$3.49
Easy-Does-It Honey Roasted Pork	**$1.02**

The estimates for my costs tend to be a little high, because I'm not sure how much a teaspoon of mustard or two tablespoons of soy sauce really costs. "Not much" seems like the right answer, but calculators don't know what to do with that kind of number.

So, how much does it cost to fill your freezer with your own frozen meals?

Using only four recipes, and spending only about 2 ½ hours total, I filled the freezer with **27 meals**, (enough for 5 ½ weeks-worth of lunches at the office!) for only **$29.22**. The same number of mass-produced meals would have cost **$88.23!**

Frankly, when I first added up these numbers, I couldn't believe I'd done it right, so I ran it through the calculator several more times. I kept coming up with the same astounding savings.

One thing that will strike you when you look at the relative costs of the individual meals is that the most expensive store-bought "healthy" meals are not the most expensive meals to make at home. The extra cost comes from branding, advertising, and luck — since some items may be on sale, and others aren't.

The other thing to remember is that your Easy-Does-It meals include healthy portions of steamed vegetables that the mass-produced meals leave out. So you get far more nutrition, better tasting meals, and higher quality food – **for about 1/3 the price!**

And it's Easy-Does-It!

Putting together an entire freezer full of meals takes very little time, especially if you create duplicates of the meals produced by the big national companies. These folks have done years of research to find the meals that will be the most satisfying while also being easy to produce for the least amount of money.

This book capitalizes on all that market research, because I've found that the entire meal, with added vegetables, can be very quickly cooked and packaged. I always do three or four different recipes, so I don't take the same thing to work every day. And one full month's of frozen meals, including shopping time, will take less than one afternoon of pleasant work.

In fact, these recipes are so easy that they're great recipes for the younger members of your family to make. It will probably take a bit longer if you have "help", but there's a definite feeling of pride (even for someone as old as me) when you see an entire freezer full of ready-to-eat meals that you made yourself. Maybe it taps into our old hunter-gatherer roots or our hording instincts.

That pride can be a great incentive for younger family members to learn to cook. And the recipes are so easy, it's almost impossible to mess any of them up.

The bean soups that you'll be putting in the freezer are especially easy to make, and are not only delicious – they are also very filling, and good for you.

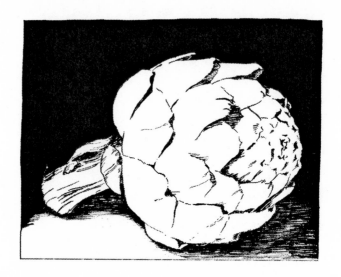

The Food

More Than Just Weight Loss

Losing weight is important, of course. But fitting into last year's jeans is not *all* that a healthy diet will do for you. By eating a low-fat, high nutrient diet you will be preparing for a longer, healthier life.

You naturally want to enjoy your life fully, and you don't want chronic disease or heart problems to slow you down. Many illnesses that bring Americans to the hospital and pharmacy are directly related to lifestyle choices, including diet. That's why it's so important to find a program that you *and your family* can follow for the long term. The Easy-Does-It Diet gives you a great start towards a lifetime of health.

There are six simple components to the Easy-Does-It Diet:

- Salads
- Steamed Vegetables

- Whole Grain Bread
- Bean Soups
- Easy-Does-It Frozen Meals
- Fruit and Fruit Smoothies

Salads

Salads are eaten for every lunch and dinner, and should be as large as you can make them. Salad greens are power-packed with fat-busting nutrition. The more you eat, the more you lose. Add a delicious low-fat, low-sugar dressing and you won't be adding extra calories or fat. We have lots of suggestions for combinations to keep you excited, but feel free to be creative.

At least once a week, you should include a small can of salmon in your salad, and occasionally add a few tablespoons of chopped raw walnuts (they are very inexpensive at Trader Joe's). This will give you the omega-3 fatty acids that protect you from heart disease.

It is almost impossible to eat too many calories if you include large portions of salads and steamed vegetables and eat only small portions of chicken or meat. The only caveat – don't pile on high-fat salad dressing, or you'll cancel out any weight-loss benefits from your salad. In fact, some restaurant Caesar salads have more calories than a Big Mac®!

You'll be starting every lunch and dinner with a salad. Make it a big one – you can't possibly eat too much. And make them festive, fun, and delicious. In fact, whenever you feel the need to "go wild" with a meal, put your creative energies into the salad. Think of those green leafy vegetables as "fat burners", and pile them on!

If you don't feel like making a fuss, then just have a simple salad – you'll still get the health-giving nutrition and fat-burning benefits, without much trouble. In fact, the new packaged salad greens include many different varieties of greens already pre-washed and ready to eat. Throw on a tomato if you want, or just add a low-cal dressing or some pineapple juice and enjoy!

Steamed Vegetables

Steamed vegetables are the easiest part of this program, after the fruit (which takes no preparation at all). Just choose pre-cut veggies in the frozen-food case at the supermarket (there's always something on sale) and divide the packages into your plastic containers.

Put them back in the freezer, and microwave them for a few minutes when you're ready to eat. I told you this was going to be easy, didn't I? You can add a dash of low-fat salad dressing for a little added zing, if you like, but the sauce on the entrée will also flavor the vegetables as your meal is being warmed in the microwave, so they always have plenty of flavor.

This diet plan emphasizes health-giving fruits and vegetables for many reasons. Weight loss may be most important to you *right at the moment*, but you'll also appreciate the fact that eating more fruits and veggies may lower your cholesterol level, and your blood pressure readings may improve. You may find you have more energy than you have in years.

Of course, all of us are different so you may not experience all these benefits – but research clearly shows that a low-fat diet that includes lots of salads, steamed vegetables, beans and fruits will help you stay healthy, and live longer – and may even help your immune system fight off disease.

Dr. Henry Mallek, an expert on nutrition and longevity, says most people believe that obesity is caused by eating more calories than we burn off with exercise.

Dr Mallek believes this is too simplistic. He believes that obesity is caused, in part, *by malnutrition*. Our bodies need many types of nutrients in order to accomplish all the millions of functions that it carries out every day. It can't do these things completely or efficiently without the help of the nutrition that we find in whole foods. Therefore, obesity is caused both by eating too many calories, and by eating *too little* of the nutrients we need.

The Easy-Does-It diet puts those nutrients back in your diet with whole grains, beans, and lots of low-calorie, high-value vegetables and greens. The added bonus is that these natural foods are filling, so you'll be able to eat more, feel full instead of deprived, and still lose weight.

Broccoli has been getting a lot of press lately because of the micro-nutrients that have been shown to add extra protection against cancer. I personally make a point of including broccoli (or one of its close relatives like cauliflower or Brussels's sprouts) in my meals at least 3 times a week. However, science has not yet discovered *all* the hidden nutrients in natural food, so be sure to eat a variety of veggies – you may get benefits that science hasn't discovered yet!

Unlike the expensive diet pills that come on the market every few years (and then get taken off the market again when they discover new health risks) you can use steamed vegetables and salads to help you lose weight without any worries about hidden risks. You'll be adding to your health, giving your body the nutrition that it needs, and reducing the calories and fat in your diet. And eating more vegetables and fruits will actually help reduce your cravings sugar, even if you're addicted to it.

Whole Grain Bread

You'll also notice that the diet includes whole grains and cereals, potatoes and brown rice. This is not a low-carb diet, but it is a low-*refined*-carb diet. Because sugar and white flour have been proven to be addictive, and many people are allergic to wheat flour without knowing it, you may feel a bit "funny" the first week or two on the diet. Sugar withdrawal symptoms can include headache, mild nausea, feeling "shaky", intestinal disturbances, or other mild physical aches and pains.

Many people mistake these symptoms for hunger pangs and give up whatever diet they're on, but this is a mistake. These mild symptoms usually last just a few days – although the addictive cravings for sugar may last far longer.

It's important to realize that sugar has been listed as one of the leading causes of the obesity epidemic by the World Health Organization. In fact, many men – who have a larger muscle mass than women (which makes weight loss easier) – may discover that the only change they need to make in order to lose their extra pounds is to leave sugar out of their diet.

This means no soda pop, no candy, no donuts, and no chocolate cake. And no processed foods that hide sugar in the ingredients. We're used to eating these items daily – but they add nothing to our nutritional needs and add unwanted pounds to our bodies. And excess sugar and other refined carbohydrates can add to your risk of getting adult-onset diabetes.

Each day you'll be eating two helpings of whole grains. Each frozen meal has ½ cup of brown rice, bulgur or whole grain pasta. If you eat a bean soup that has no whole grain included in the recipe, you will eat a slice of whole grain bread with your soup.

Whole grain bread is not as easy to find as you would think. I've checked the ingredients list of several dark-looking breads at the store, and the first ingredient is almost always 'wheat flour'. Don't be fooled into believing they mean 'whole wheat flour'. They don't.

Most dark wheat bread is just white bread with some caramel coloring added. Some of them include whole wheat flour in the ingredients to add flavor, but white flour makes up the largest part of the bread. White flour gives you almost no nutrition, but it gives you lots of calories. It's the last thing you need when you're trying to lose weight.

H. E. Jacob, the author of *Six Thousand Years of Bread: Its Holy and Unholy History* wrote this back in 1944: "What a strange, fortuitous course does the history of man pursue. The technological crisis of the Middle Ages made men eat splinters of stone in their flour; the technological progress of our industrial age has produced machines so precise that they grind away the living strength of the flour." This shows that it has been known for over half a century that white flour has no nutritional value, except for the few nutrients that must be added back in, by law.

Real whole wheat bread is fun to bake yourself, but most of us don't have time. If you have a spare afternoon, I strongly suggest that you try it, because the kneading and baking of whole-grain bread is a wonderfully creative experience.

I have found that whole wheat tortillas can usually be found in the local supermarket. (I like to crisp mine in the microwave for about a minute, and eat it like a large cracker. I like to watch them puff up as they heat, but be careful to not let them burn.) I also have found whole wheat and other whole grain dinner rolls and pita breads at Trader Joe's. You may have a bakery nearby that makes low-fat, low-sugar whole wheat bread. Just be sure to check the labels.

Please don't make the mistake of thinking that one of those giant bran muffins or huge bagels at the local coffee-shop and Costco's will equal a slice of whole grain bread. For one thing, they're at least three times bigger than a slice of bread, and the muffins include lots of sugar and butter or other oil. Think of them as very large donuts without the hole. Just because they add some bran doesn't mean they're good for you. And almost all bagels are made primarily from white flour, which is not included on this diet.

If you're in the habit of grabbing one of these monsters for breakfast, you'll have to give it up or be resigned to staying overweight.

If you find that you aren't losing weight as quickly as you would like (1 pound a week is considered reasonable after the initial week), bread (and pasta) are components of this diet that you should leave out. You can add them back into your diet when you've reached your ideal weight.

Many people find that they feel better when they don't eat wheat bread or pasta, and they feel less bloated – probably because they have a hidden allergy to wheat. This is the part of the diet that you'll need to fiddle with until you find what's best for your own body. Brown rice pasta has a very nice, subtle flavor, and is a very good substitute for the white flour pasta your family is probably used to.

Easy-Does-It Frozen Meals

The frozen meals with meat all contain about 3 oz. of chicken or other flesh food, or a bean entrée, along with a tasty sauce or gravy, plus ½ cup of whole grain such as brown rice, bulgur, or whole grain noodles, and lots of frozen vegetables. The recipes are easy to do, and you'll be able to put three different entrées and a bean soup in the freezer in just a few hours.

This storehouse of nutrition will last you for several weeks — all cooking and cleanup are done just once, and you never have to think about what to eat next. Just cook another entrée when you have six empty containers, and you'll continue to add to the variety in your freezer.

The portions of meat and whole grains are important because these are concentrated foods. But portion control is easy — because you'll be making the meals long in advance, when you aren't hungry.

There are two kinds of Easy-Does-It frozen meals — Some have meat and some have beans. You will be eating beans (*"the dieter's best friend"*) at least once a day. I suggest that you eat your beans at lunch, because the slowly digesting carbohydrates and proteins in the beans will keep you from getting the mid-afternoon munchies.

You'll soon find that beans are incredibly versatile. To make it easy, choose a meal with beans for lunch, and a meal with meat for dinner. That way you'll have the meat you like each day, and the beans that help you lose weight. (I personally prefer the meals with beans, and usually choose them far more often than once a day – if you don't want to eat the meat you certainly don't have to.)

I'm absolutely amazed that the bean, one of the most nutritious foods we can eat, is also one of the least expensive! There are many people in this country who refuse to eat beans because they don't cost enough money – how silly can you get?

Many traditional peoples in all parts of the world rely heavily on beans in their diet. When food is scarce, and doctors are a long ways away and far too expensive, people place the greatest emphasis on foods that keep them healthy. In Asia people have soy and mung beans, in Central and South America people rely on black and kidney beans, and the Mediterranean cultures have fava beans and chickpeas. Here in America we have access to all of them and hundreds of other varieties. But we don't eat them nearly enough.

The Adventist Health study, undertaken by the Loma Linda University in Southern California, looked at the connection between diet and colon cancer. They found that individuals who ate beans at least two times a week had a 42 percent lower risk of developing colon cancer than those who said they ate beans less than once a week. The same study found that eating tomatoes and beans (a natural combination) gave some protection against prostrate cancer.

According to Dr. Joe Fuhrman, beans can stabilize blood sugar, reduce your desire for sugary food, and prevent mid-afternoon cravings. He believes that beans should be considered your best friend if you're on a diet.

Beans are so important in the Easy-Does-It Diet that you'll be having them at least once a day. Don't worry – there are so many varieties and so many ways of preparing them that you won't get bored. If you're worried about the gas that sometimes comes after we eat beans, just buy some Beano. It works.

Fruit

Your fruit will be eaten at every breakfast, and for snacks. You can always find a variety of fruit at your local market.

The Asian supermarket in our city has a fantastic variety of fruit, and it always feels like an adventure to shop there. For some reason their prices are lower than the big chain stores, too. We also have a farmer's market that comes every Saturday, selling local fruit from outlying farms. And berry patches are dotted around the area, even in the suburbs. They put signs out when the fruit is ripe.

If you can find farms that let you pick your own, it makes a wonderful outing for the family. Children always love a trip to the farm, even when it's just down the street. The fruit is usually less expensive, too, when you pick your own. You can freeze anything you can't eat right away.

Included in the fruit category are delicious fruit smoothies that you'll make with frozen fruit, skim milk or light soymilk, and a touch of honey. These smoothies are wonderful for breakfast or deserts, and your kids will love them as much as you do.

Humans crave sweet things because we need the nutrients in fruit and sweet vegetables. Unfortunately, in the last 50 years or so many of us have been feeding our appetite for sweetness by eating way too much sugar.

Sugar is an un-natural, highly refined substance that is mined from cane and beets — and all the nutrients from those plants are thrown away! Sugar will alter your insulin reaction, cause you to gain weight, increase your chances of becoming diabetic, and can even affect your mood. The book *Sugar Blues*, by William F. Dufty, was first written in 1975, so the dangers of sugar have been known for years.

But what do you do eat if you don't eat sugar? *You eat fruit.* After all, that's what your body is asking for when it tells you it wants something sweet. Eat a piece of fruit for breakfast, for mid-meal snacks, and for desert. Your body will love you for it.

And what do you drink if you need to stay away from sugar? Instead of diet drinks, which include artificial sweeteners, and instead of fruit juices, which contain far too much fructose and no fiber, I suggest water, green tea, herbal teas, or bouillon that has been made without added salt. It's important to get enough water, and equally important to stay away from sugar. Try a variety of hot and cold drinks throughout the day, and find the ones that you most enjoy.

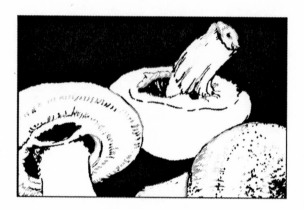

Behavior Modification

Breaking Old Habits

One of the biggest obstacles to successful weight loss comes from our own habits – we cook and eat today what we cooked and ate last week, and last year. Unfortunately, most Americans habitually eat the wrong food – or too much of it. And we get fat.

To put it bluntly, losing weight requires *behavior modification*. That means we have to change the way we act and make different choices. We might wish for a magic pill that will take away our excess fat without taking away the fattening food, but it isn't going to happen in our lifetime.

And forget the magic potato chips deep-fried in anti-fat – what you need is *healthy* food, not artificial substitutes for unhealthy food. You already know that.

However, the **Easy-Does-It Diet** makes change easy, by providing delicious, ready-made meals and simple menu plans. You can stay committed to your diet and health goals while concentrating on other things in life that are more interesting and fun.

You probably also know that you'll lose weight faster if you increase the exercise you get each day. Walk briskly at least 20 minutes a day, or join an aerobics class at the gym. Get out in the fresh air and play with your kids or your dog. Do something!

Recent research has also shown that adding strength training to your weekly exercise routine can help even more than aerobic exercise. You do burn fat while you're walking, but the firmer muscles you get from lifting light weights will let you burn fat even while you're resting or watching TV.

Most men have an unfair advantage over women when it comes to losing weight – they have bigger muscles, so just a small increase in exercise or a small decrease in calorie consumption will help most men return to their ideal weight. Women have smaller muscles, but if you start a simple weight lifting program you will improve your metabolism dramatically and tone your body at the same time.

If you have fibromyalgia, back pain, or any other condition that makes exercise difficult or painful, you should discuss this with your doctor. She may be able to find specific exercises that will work for you, or she may have recommendations that will allow you to lose weight in spite of your inactivity. If you and your doctor believe that you have different dietary needs, you can still use the basic ideas behind this book, but add your own variations as needed.

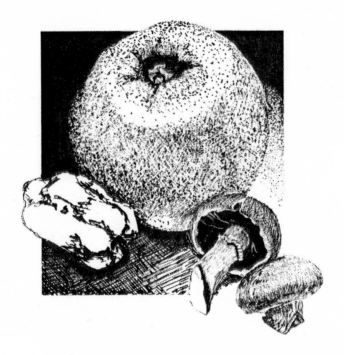

Getting Ready

Equipment You'll Need

To use this diet, you'll need access to a freezer. The freezer that comes with your refrigerator is perfectly adequate. However, if you're like most of us, your freezer may already be crammed full. Just take a few minutes to rearrange the contents so that you'll have room for the Easy-Does-It Diet meals you'll be creating this weekend.

You'll also need access to a microwave oven, preferably for both lunch and dinner. If you don't have a microwave that you can use at work, you can still use this diet. Just take a full-meal salad, which includes cooked canned beans or salmon, or frozen peas, and whole-grain pasta. Just be sure to make it a big salad so you don't get hungry in the afternoon

You'll need a stovetop and cooking pans, of course. And for the frozen fruit smoothies, you'll need a blender.

Making it Easy

You'll need to set aside a weekend afternoon to shop for your ingredients and to fill your freezer with healthy, delicious meals. To make your project as efficient as possible, you'll want to choose two, three or four recipes to cook in one afternoon.

The recipes in the book include a shopping list, so you'll have a handy reference when you're preparing to shop. Many of the ingredients will already be on your pantry shelves.

To begin the process you'll need to purchase some plastic containers. My favorites are the Glad Ware® and Ziploc® containers, entrée (3 1/8 cups) and short round (1 ¾ cups) sizes. The smaller containers, which you'll use for your bean soups, can be a little difficult to find. You might also want to use the divided entrée containers that they've just come out with, so that you can have a meal with the juicier bean soups without having to take two different containers.

You'll also need at least one plastic container for your salads, to hold at least 4 cups.

The containers can be used over and over, but are not expensive. I found the entrée size Glad Ware containers on sale at the local Fred Meyer's for $2.00 a package, with 5 containers and lids in the package. For $8 I had enough for 20 frozen meals. You'll only need to buy them once (unless you lose them, of course.)

If you balk at the initial cost, remember that frozen meals from the supermarket add the cost of the container and packaging to *every* meal you buy. With the Easy-Does-It system, you only have to pay for the containers once.

If you allow your lunch to thaw in the refrigerator or at your desk during the morning, they will only take 1 ½ to 2 minutes to microwave at lunch-time. If you keep your lunch in the freezer at work, they will take approximately 4 ½ to 5 minutes. You'll need to experiment a little, since all microwaves are a little different.

When you're packaging your meals in your Glad Ware® containers, you'll notice that the entrée and grain or potatoes will take up about i/4 of the space. Fill the rest with your favorite frozen vegetable. Don't cook the vegetables first — just open the bag and pour them into the container beside the entrée and the potatoes or rice, then throw them in the freezer.

Much of your nutrition will come from these veggies, so don't skimp! There are almost no calories in steamed vegetables, but there are tons of micro-nutrients that your body needs. And they help you feel full, which helps you stay away from the candy machine.

Not Just for Dieting

I can actually think of many times when a freezer full of complete, light meals would be useful. The obvious is for evenings when you just don't feel like cooking. Long after you've lost your excess weight, you'll want to keep a supply of ready-made, healthy meals in your freezer.

When you have a hard day at work, there's no need to stop for groceries or pizza, because you have a complete, healthy meal that will be ready in just a few minutes. And your kids will appreciate having a meal ready for them whenever you'll be late getting home.

The Easy-Does-It light meals are the perfect size for older folks, too, who often don't get enough variety in their diets if they have to cook for themselves. Most mass-produced frozen meals don't include enough vegetables to keep you at optimum health, and they cost too much for many seniors on fixed budgets.

And one other thing our family discovered after our grandfather had a stroke – there are no packaged meals that can be opened with one hand. Glad Ware containers are much easier to open, but they do get hot in the microwave, and the steam escaping from the lid can burn. Caution is needed when removing them from the oven.

If you have an older family member on a fixed income who needs the convenience of packaged meals, but who needs more nutrition and an easier package, you can fill her freezer with Easy-Does-It meals for less than $30. If she eats two meals a day, this will be enough for two full weeks, and the entire freezer can be filled with just a few hours work. Add some packaged salad greens and low fat dressing and your older loved one will be getting all the nutrition she needs to stay healthy and alert. With some creativity, special diets can be easily accommodated.

Flexibility

If you find yourself getting hungry, increase your helping of salad or steamed vegetables. You can't eat too much of these foods, and many experts really believe that the *more you eat, the more you'll lose.* Some people even call them "negative calorie" foods. What a wonderful idea –

there's no excuse for feeling deprived or picked on because you can literally eat as much as you want.

If you live with a family, you can use this plan in two different ways. You can fix one recipe for dinner, add a large salad, and share with everyone – just make sure you pay attention to portion control when you serve yourself the meat, rice, bread, potatoes or pasta. With the salad and the veggies you can eat as much as you want.

Or you may find it's easier to stay on track by cooking your family their "regular" meal, and then pulling your own meal from the freezer to microwave just before the family's meal is ready to serve. If you aren't the one who cooks the evening meal, this may be the best option, because you won't need to convince the rest of the family that they need to make changes in *their diet* in order to help you lose weight.

Shopping for Your Salad

Salads can contain as many different varieties of fresh raw veggies as you want – or you can just add a tomato to some romaine lettuce and add some low-fat salad dressing. Some weeks you'll feel like going wild, other times you'll just want to get in the store and out again. Try to make things as simple as possible, but still make sure that you're getting enough variety to stay interested.

A friend of mine absolutely swears by Weight Watcher's®, a diet plan that also lets you eat as much salad as you want. Unfortunately, she didn't build her salad at home and bring it to work so she was limited to the only salad available for sale in the restaurant near her office. She ate the same salad every day for several months, and gave up her diet out of sheer boredom and regained the extra weight.

So get creative, but don't get carried away. If you see some veggies at the market that look really enticing, throw them in your shopping cart. You don't need to follow our salad recipes exactly, as long as you eat your salad.

I've found that the very best, most nutritious base for a salad is the pre-washed packaged salad greens available in most supermarkets. Some of the packages include mesclun mixes that include such tasty greens as lettuce, kale, chard, mustard, arugula, and many more. The variety multiplies the fat-burning nutrients in your salad.

They seem a bit expensive, but the convenience in this case seems worth it to me. You can have a variety of greens without filling your refrigerator drawer, and you can buy just what you need so they don't wilt and get thrown out.

Another excellent option is to grow your own greens. Many people don't realize that the most nutritious foods we can eat, the salad greens, are also some of the easiest foods to grow. They aren't fond of summer heat, but many of the varieties of lettuce and other greens can winter over in a protected greenhouse. And you can even grow some in containers on your deck.

If you have a little extra room, or if you're already planning a garden, I strongly suggest that you check out the mesclun mixes at Johnny's Seeds. You can find them on the Internet at http://www.johnnyseeds.com

Breakfast

To make sure that you have enough fruit each day, you'll want to start out with fruit for breakfast. This not only makes breakfast incredibly easy (how hard can it be to peel a banana?) but you'll also be helping to stabilize your blood sugar, making it less likely that you'll feel a compulsive need to eat a candy bar at mid-morning break.

Have two or more pieces of breakfast every morning. You can choose from strawberries, bananas, oranges, grapefruit, raspberries – you name it. It's an easy, nutritious way to start your day.

Several times a week you may want to have a small bowl of oatmeal or shredded wheat. Oatmeal has been shown to lower your cholesterol, and helps you feel full. It's also a great way to warm up on a cold morning, and a nice steaming bowl of oatmeal makes many people feel cared for – because most of us grew up with oatmeal when we were kids. Please note - I'm actually talking about *oatmeal* here – not the sugared, refined, packaged and discombobulated stuff they sell as flavored "instant" oatmeal.

The best oatmeal (in my opinion) is the Snoqualmie Falls® brand, which can be found in many supermarkets next to the big round Quaker Oats® boxes. Snoqualmie Falls oatmeal has more body to it, and doesn't get mushy when it's cooked. I love the texture, and the flavor is superior to the other brands. If you tell yourself you really don't like oatmeal, you should give Snoqualmie Falls oatmeal a try. It's a bit more expensive, but it's worth it if you actually eat the stuff.

Add a banana or a small amount of currants or raisins, and some non-fat milk. You now have a simple, easy-to-prepare breakfast for the days when you have time to sit down and eat. For most days of the week, however, you should have one or two pieces of fruit.

About fruit juice — it isn't included in this plan. Fruit juice is concentrated fructose, a natural form of sugar. It's high in calories, and it goes directly to your bloodstream, causing spikes in your blood sugar levels. This can disrupt your insulin response, and also leads to sugar cravings around 10am.

The fiber in whole fruit prevents the sugar spike from happening, so you can get the full nutritional value from the fruit without the weight gain and cravings caused by fruit juice. The only exception will be the fruit juice you use as flavorings in salad dressings and other recipes.

This breakfast chapter is very short, because breakfast should be very simple. One or two pieces of fruit, or a small bowl of oatmeal with fruit and skim milk. **Never leave out the fruit.** This diet plan gives your body the nutrients it needs in order to become more efficient, and it needs the nutrients in fruit to function properly. Don't even think about telling me you don't have time for breakfast!

Between Meal Snacks

Fruit. Apples, plums, apricots, grapes, watermelon, peaches, bananas, oranges, kumquats....

You'll be eating one or two pieces of fruit to get you started in the morning, and by mid-morning break you'll be ready for another piece of fruit. Have another piece of fruit in the mid-afternoon. Be sure to pick up a nice variety of easy-to-carry fruit when you do the weekly shopping.

The meal plans all include fruit for lunch and dinner, but you won't need to eat additional fruit if you've already had your four pieces during the day as snacks. The fruit smoothies are great for breakfast or for a quick pick-me-up when you get home from work. Fit the fruit in the way that's most convenient for you.

Many families think of fruit as a luxury that they can't afford. This is only true if you focus on meat in your meals. Meat is truly expensive, considering the amount of nutrition you get per pound. Fruit is always comparatively less expensive than meat and far more nutritious, but our 'normal' American diet leaves it out. Big mistake.

Have you ever seen a small child in a strawberry patch? Then you know that humans instinctively reach for fruit.

The best fruit is fresh, and there's almost always something on sale. Farmer's markets are great because you know the fruit is fresh and you will be supporting your local farmers. And many homes have fruit trees in the backyard that never get picked. Get creative, and enjoy!

Canned fruit has sugar added in most cases, and should be avoided. Frozen fruit, such as strawberries and blueberries, are very convenient for adding to your morning oatmeal.

One very large benefit that comes from spending the money on fruit instead of expensive meat is that your children will be less apt to become addicted to sugar. Children love fruit, and this is really what their little bodies are craving when their appetites lead them to sweet food. In America we usually hand children candy instead of fruit, but that leads to a lot of problems later on.

Sugar is bad for the teeth and it causes children to become obese – which in turn adds to their risk of diabetes. And overweight children have a much harder time fitting in at school. If you get in the habit of adding plenty of fruit to your own diet, it will be much easier to remember to provide fruit for your kids, as well.

At the beginning, when you are looking for faster weight loss, you may want to keep snacking to a minimum, and have only two or three pieces of fruit each day. It is possible to slow down your weight loss by eating too much fruit, and if this happens, just substitute raw vegetables as snacks until you reach your weight loss goal.

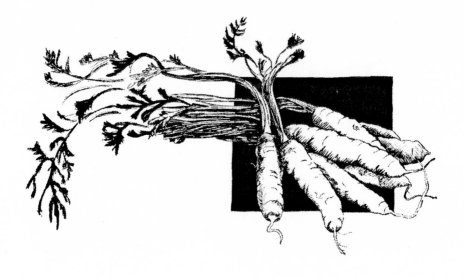

Easy-Does-It Frozen Meals

Each week's meal plan includes seven Easy-Does-It frozen meals with meat, and seven meals with beans. You won't need to cook 14 different recipes, since each recipe fills six entrée containers. Choose two meat dishes and two bean dishes to start with, and then cook and freeze another batch as soon as you have six empty containers. That way you will be constantly refreshing the stock in your freezer, and you'll end up with enough variety to keep yourself interested.

On the day that I wrote this chapter I got home from the supermarket around noon. I cooked four recipes — Pasta with Beans and Pesto, Barley and White Bean Stew, Chicken Alfredo, and Chicken Adobo. By 2:30 all the pans were in the dishwasher, 24 delicious meals were in the freezer, and I was back at my computer.

The best thing about this plan, in my mind, is the fact that I won't have to clean up after my messy cooking for almost two weeks! And I cooked this batch before the freezer was empty, so I have several other varieties still waiting for me. There will be plenty to choose from this week, and I won't get bored.

To save money on the meat dishes I buy the frozen, skinned, boneless chicken breast in the 4 pound packages. You can almost always find them on sale for about $8.00. This is enough chicken for 4 complete recipes, more than a month's worth of evening meals! The one drawback to this plan is that the chicken breasts have water added, making browning almost impossible. I just leave out the browning step, but it does cut down on the flavor. You can also find other cuts of meat in 'family' packs that are considerably less costly per pound than buying small amounts at a time.

Of course, the bean dishes are all so inexpensive that you won't have to worry about cost, even though you'll be using cooked, canned beans to save time.

You will need to purchase frozen vegetables to put in the containers with your entrées. You'll want about 2 pounds for every recipe – but every brand comes in a different sized bag. Once you've become used to eating this many vegetables, you'll get used to eyeballing the packages in the store, and knowing how many containers they'll fill.

Remember, the suggestions that I include for vegetables are just that – suggestions. Buy whatever vegetables you know you love, and whatever happens to be on sale. They're all good for you! Just don't get the kind that already has sauce or pasta included. These products are much more expensive, and include items that are not on your diet. Stick with the plain-Jane veggies – but do take advantage of the wonderful assortment of mixed vegetables that are now available.

Also remember all the good things they're saying about the health benefits of broccoli, and include this delicious vegetable, or its close cousins such as cauliflower or Brussels sprouts, as often as possible.

.You can add even more variety by using two different kinds of vegetables for every entrée recipe. If you do two different entrée recipes, this will give you four different meals for the same amount of time and trouble. Or put both kinds of vegetables in each container – it's totally up to you. Be creative.

After looking over the recipes you'll probably notice two things – first, these are not gourmet recipes. They are actually chosen to be closest to what mom would have cooked, so that you won't have to make too many changes in your life all at once. Second, you'll immediately think of your own favorite recipes that can be used for the Easy-Does-It Diet frozen meals. Use these recipes only as a starting place.

How to Use Your Own Favorite Recipes

You can see from looking at the recipes in this book that they are simply old family favorites, converted to low-fat versions, and portioned in a specific way in their individual containers. I didn't have room in this book to include every possible recipe, and I know I've left out a few of your favorites. Here's how to turn your own special recipes into an Easy-Does-It frozen meal:

If your recipe includes chicken, pork or beef, make sure you begin with approximately 18 oz of meat, just a smidge over 1 pound. When your recipe is cooked and divided into six plastic freezer containers, each container will have no more than 3 oz. of meat. If your recipe uses sausage or another high-fat meat, reduce the amount you begin with to ¾ pound, and be sure to pour off any extra fat that renders out during browning.

If your recipe includes pasta of any kind, use whole grain pasta. The whole grain pasta that tastes most like 'normal' pasta is made from brown rice, and can be found in natural food stores. You can also find it online at some whole-foods websites. I did some surfing and found some at an online store called Village Organics, at http://www.villageorganics.com/browricfusor.html

Both meat and grains are concentrated foods, and that means that you need to carefully portion your pasta as well as your meat. 1 oz will make approximately ½ cup of cooked pasta, so you'll need 6 oz to fill six containers. Since all pasta comes in different sized packages, you may need to do some guessing. But don't get carried away, as most Americans do, and give yourself a huge portion of pasta – unless you're really resigned to being overweight.

If your recipe has potatoes or rice, barley, corn, or bulgur, use the ½ cup cooked grain per container rule.

No matter what recipe you use for your entrée, it should fill about ¼ of your container, and the rest should be filled with frozen, cut-up vegetables. Use the veggies you love, or whatever happens to be on sale. For the sake of your health, include broccoli as often as possible. Don't cook the veggies – simply add them to the container and throw them back in the freezer. They'll cook in the microwave while your entrée is warming up.

Fats and oils should be kept to a minimum. To do that, choose low-fat cuts of meat, and keep your meat portions at 3 oz or less. Pour off any extra fat that renders out during cooking. To sauté vegetables, use one tablespoon olive oil, use a non-stick spray, or sauté with two tablespoons of water instead of oil.

For most recipes that call for a lot of oil, you can use far less than your recipe calls for and still have a very flavorful dish. Some recipes depend on very large amounts of butter or olive oil for flavor – if they won't taste right without the gobs of fat and oil, cook something else.

What About Left-overs?

Some left-overs are perfect for Easy-Does-It Diet frozen meals. Pot-roast with potatoes, for instance, could easily be portioned into 3 oz pieces of meat and ½ cup of potatoes. Just be careful of your portions, and give yourself plenty of veggies. Remember to eat one bean dish each day, either for lunch or dinner. Your favorite chili recipe, if you watch the amount of meat that you use, would be perfect for this diet.

Some bean soup recipes call for salt pork or ham hocks. Others, such as Boston Baked Beans, also call for large amounts of molasses, maple syrup, or sugar. Please use your judgment – you can often add the traditional flavor with a little bit of bacon, crisped and then drained of fat. Sometimes the dish is just as good without the salted fat added. I generally choose another recipe. It's often easier than making myself believe I'm not missing the flavors I've grown to expect in high-fat, high-salt, high-sugar foods.

I hope you find the following recipes tasty and easy to prepare.

Sweet and Sour Chicken

With rice and green peas

Recipe makes 6 frozen meals. This recipe can be used with either white or brown rice. The brown rice will add more nutrients, with fewer calories. Check the rice package for cooking directions.

Shopping list:

1 8 oz. can unsweetened pineapple chunks in their own juice (Trader Joe's sells chunked fresh pineapple in its own juice, but canned is fine if it has no added sugar)
1 1/4 lb boneless, skinless chicken breast
1 can non-fat chicken broth
1 green pepper
1 red or orange pepper
2 1-lb package frozen peas or pea pods
1 onion

Staples:

Vinegar
Honey
Cornstarch
Soy sauce
Brown rice

Recipe:

In a small saucepan mix the following:

1/2 cup pineapple juice
1/4 cup chicken broth or water
3 Tablespoons vinegar
1 Tablespoon honey
1 Tablespoons soy sauce
1 Tablespoon corn starch

Cook sauce until it thickens slightly, and becomes clear. Set aside.

Cut **1 ¼ lb boneless, skinless chicken breast** into 3/4 inch cubes. Cut **½ onion** into ½ inch chunks.

Spray a wok or large skillet with non-stick spray or add 2 tablespoons olive or canola oil. Brown the chicken pieces.

Add the sauce and onion pieces to the chicken, and simmer, covered, for about ½ hour or until chicken chunks are tender.

While the chicken is cooking, place **1 cup brown rice** in rice cooker or medium sauce pan. Add 1 ½ to 2 cups of water (depending on package directions) and pinch of salt if desired. Add lid and cook until rice is done, about 45 minutes.

When chicken is tender, uncover and allow to cool. When mixture has cooled add:

¾ cup drained pineapple chunks
1 green pepper and
1 red or orange pepper, seeds and membranes removed, cut into ½ inch chunks.

Do not cook after vegetables and pineapple have been added. They will cook when the lunch is heated in the microwave.

Spoon rice, evenly divided, into 6 entrée sized containers. (Keep your rice in one corner of the container) Open **2 packages of green peas or pea pods** and pour into containers. Add chicken-pineapple mixture on top of rice. Add lids, making sure seal is tight. Place containers in freezer.

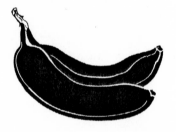

Honey Glazed Pork

With roasted potatoes and broccoli

Recipe makes six frozen meals.
Shopping list:

1 lb pork chops, boneless
2 lbs baby red potatoes
2 1-lb packages frozen broccoli

Staples:

Honey
Soy sauce
Prepared mustard

Recipe:

In small bowl combine:

¼ cup honey
¼ cup soy sauce
1 teaspoon prepared mustard

Cut 3 lbs of baby red potatoes into halves or quarters, making all pieces approximately the same size.

Spray large skillet with non-stick spray or coat with olive or canola oil. Add pork chops and brown. Add baby potatoes and honey mustard sauce, and cover over low heat.

Allow chops and potatoes to cook until pork is tender, approximately 45 minutes to 1 hour, depending on thickness of meat. Stir potatoes occasionally to coat with sauce.

When meat is tender, remove from heat and allow to cool slightly. Divide meat and potatoes evenly between six entrée sized containers. Add frozen broccoli (do not cook broccoli before placing in containers. The vegetable will cook when the lunch is heated in the microwave.

Place containers in freezer.

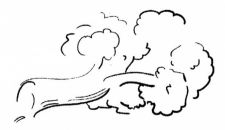

Herbed Chicken

With spicy roasted potatoes and mixed vegetables

The roasted potato recipe below is for those who like hot, spicy food. To tone it down, just reduce or eliminate the hot oil.

Shopping list:

1 ¼ lb boneless, skinless chicken breast
2 lb Yukon gold potatoes
2 1-lb package frozen mixed vegetables
1 can non-fat cream of chicken soup

Staples:

Herbs (Mrs. Dash or mixture to your taste)
Olive oil
Hot pepper sauce or oil (optional)

Recipe:

Heat oven to 350°.

Cut Yukon gold potatoes into bite-sized chunks. In small bowl mix together:

¼ cup olive oil
2 tablespoons hot pepper sauce (Tabasco) or pepper oil (optional)
1 teaspoon freshly ground black pepper
1 to 2 teaspoons herb mixture (Mrs. Dash Extra Spicy or to your own mixture, to taste)

Place potatoes in bottom of roasting pan, and pour oil/herb mixture over them. Stir to coat evenly. Roast in oven until potatoes are tender, about 45 minutes.

Cut **1 ¼ lb chicken** into 6 equal pieces. Spray large skillet with non-stick spray or add 1 tablespoon olive or canola oil. Brown chicken. Add **1 can of cream of chicken soup,** and **1 to 2 teaspoons herb mixture**. (Mrs. Dash or to your taste.) Add lid and cook over medium low heat until chicken is tender and sauce is creamy, about 45 minutes. Remove from heat and allow to cool slightly.

When potatoes are tender, you can brown them slightly under the broiler, if you like. Remove from oven and allow to cool slightly.

Add chicken to containers, and cover with sauce. Add potatoes and **2 package2 mixed frozen vegetables**. Place in freezer.

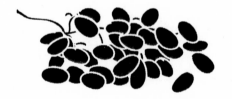

Chicken "Alfredo" with Vegetables

With parmesan cheese sauce

Recipe makes 6 frozen entrees. You can actually get creative and leave out the chicken – it's still delicious!

Shopping list:

1 ¼ lb chicken breast, skinless and boneless
1 can non-fat cream of chicken soup
2 1 lb packages mixed vegetables with asparagus
1 8 oz package penne pasta (or whatever shape you like)
4 oz grated parmesan or parmesan/Romano blend

Staples:

Pepper

Recipe:

Cut **1 ¼ lbs chicken** breast into ¾ inch chunks. Spray large skillet or wok with non-stick spray or add 1 tablespoon olive or canola oil. Brown chicken for about 5 minutes, until golden.

Add **1 can non-fat cream of chicken soup** and cover. Cook over low heat until chicken is tender, 45 minutes to 1 hour. Remove from heat.

In the meantime, cook **pasta** according to package directions in a large pot. Drain.

Add cooked chicken and sauce to the pasta pan, and add:

2 packages frozen mixed vegetables with asparagus
4 oz parmesan or parmesan/Romano blend.

Add **pepper** to taste. Mix thoroughly and divide between
6 containers.

Mixture will look strange because the cheese has not
melted. Vegetables will cook and cheese will melt when
the meals are heated in microwave.

Place containers in freezer.

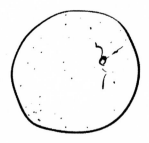

Salisbury Steak

With garlic mashed potatoes and mushroom gravy

This recipe makes six meals. If your coworkers won't let you get away with the garlic in the mashed potatoes, simply leave it out. They'll still be good.

Shopping list:

1 to 1 ¼ lb lean ground beef
8 oz mushrooms
1 16 oz can non-fat beef broth, un-condensed
6 medium potatoes
1 small can non-fat chicken broth
Garlic
1 package frozen mixed vegetables

Staples:

Corn starch
Salt and pepper

Recipe:

Peel 6 medium potatoes and cut into quarters. Place in saucepan and cover with water. If desired, add 4 peeled, whole cloves of garlic. Bring water to a boil, and cover. Simmer potatoes for about 15 minutes, or until tender.

While potatoes are simmering, slice the wash and slice the mushrooms, and place in small saucepan. Reserve ¼ cup of the 16 oz can of non-fat beef broth. Pour the remaining broth over mushrooms and bring to a simmer, and gently cook for about 10 to 15 minutes, until mushrooms are tender.

Divide 1 lb ground beef into 6 patties, approximately ½ inch thick. Spray broiler pan with non-stick spray or coat lightly with olive or canola oil. Place patties under broiler, about 6 inches below heating element. Broil for approximately 6 minutes on each side, until cooked through and lightly browned.
Drain water from potatoes, and add salt and pepper to taste. Pour in ¼ to ½ cup chicken broth as you mash the potatoes by hand or with electric mixer.

Place one patty in each of six containers, and divide mashed potatoes evenly between them, making a slight indentation in potatoes.

Add one tablespoon of cornstarch to reserved beef broth, and stir till completely combined. Add slowly to simmering mushroom sauce, stirring continually. Continue to simmer until sauce regains its dark brown color and is clear. Add pepper to taste. (Most beef broth is pre-salted).

Pour mushroom gravy over hamburger patty and potatoes. Add frozen mixed vegetables, cover, and place in freezer.

Chicken Adobo

With string beans and carrots

This is a very flavorful meal that gets you away from the blah feeling that sometimes comes with a diet. You can actually leave the chicken out.

Shopping list:

1 1/4 pound skinned, boneless chicken breast or pork
2 or 3 large carrots
2 medium potatoes
2 green or red sweet peppers
2 medium onions
½ package frozen string beans

Staples:

Garlic
Pepper
Bay leaves
Soy sauce
Vinegar

To cook:

Cut 1 ¼ lb. **chicken breast** or **lean pork** into ¾ inch cubes. Add meat to medium sauce pan, along with 2 cloves **garlic**, finely chopped, ¼ teaspoon **pepper**, 2 **bay leaves**, ½ cup **soy sauce** (low salt if available), ½ cup **vinegar**, and 1 cup water.

Simmer until meat is almost tender, about 30 minutes. Meanwhile, cut into large pieces:

2 – 3 large carrots
2 medium potatoes
2 green or red sweet peppers
2 medium yellow onions

Place carrots, potatoes and onions in the pot with the chicken, and simmer for about 15 minutes. Add the sweet peppers and ½ package string beans, and continue cooking, covered, until vegetables are tender-crisp.

Stir 2 tablespoons cornstarch with a little water, and slowly add to broth, stirring constantly, until broth becomes clear and slightly thick. Remove from heat.

Divide Chicken Adobo evenly into 6 plastic containers, and 2 packages frozen mixed vegetables. Add lids, and place in freezer.

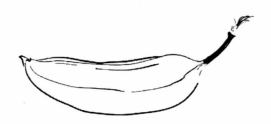

Potato Curry with Peas

With broccoli

This recipe has peas, a legume, and can be used in any meal that calls for bean soup.

Shopping list:

1 package of frozen green peas
2 medium baking potatoes or 1 lb new yellow potatoes
2 onions
2 large tomatoes
1 package frozen broccoli
Parsley
Lemon
2 small green chilies (optional)

Staples:

Salt
Garam masala and turmeric (or curry powder)
Garlic
Brown rice

Recipe:

Place 1 cup **brown rice** and 1 ½ cup water (or to package directions) in medium saucepan or rice steamer. Bring to simmer, cover, and cook over low heat for about 40 minutes, or until done.

Add about one tablespoon of water to a heavy fry pan and add 1 **onion**, finely chopped and 2 cloves of **garlic**, crushed and chopped. Water-sauté the onion and garlic until soft but not brown over medium high heat.

Add:

>2 large tomatoes, chopped
>¾ teaspoon garam masala
>¾ teaspoon ground turmeric
>(or substitute one to three teaspoons of mild curry powder for the two spices above)
>½ teaspoon salt
>2 fresh green chilies, chopped (optional)
>2 tablespoons fresh parsley, chopped

Stir-fry for 2 to 3 minutes, until tomatoes are soft. Add 2 tablespoons of **water**, 1 Tablespoon **lemon juice**, 2 **medium potatoes or 1 lb. new yellow** potatoes, cubed.

Cover the pan loosely and slowly simmer, stirring occasionally, until the sauce is thick and the potatoes are tender. Add a little more water during cooking, if needed.

When potatoes are tender, remove from heat and cool slightly. Add on 1 lb. package frozen peas to potato mixture, and gently stir. Do not cook after peas are added, or they'll be too mushy after re-heating.

When rice is done, divide evenly between six plastic entrée containers. Add Potato Curry with Peas, and fill remainder of container with frozen broccoli. Place lids on containers, and place in freezer.

Arroz con Pollo (Chicken with Rice)

With peas

This recipe combines the chicken and sauce with the rice, so it's very flavorful and easy to cook.

Shopping list:

1 ¼ lb chicken breast, boneless and skinless
1 onion
1 green or red pepper
Celery
Small can of tomato paste
1 can chicken broth
1 8 oz pkg frozen peas
2 1 lb packages frozen vegetables
Lemon

Staples:

Garlic
Cumin
Oregano
Pepper
Brown rice

Recipe:

Cut chicken breast in ½ inch chunks and sprinkle with pepper to taste, and juice from ½ lemon. Brown in large saucepan with 1 tablespoon of olive oil. Remove chicken and set aside.

To hot oil in saucepan add:

> ½ onion, chopped
> 1 green or rep pepper, chopped
> 1 to 2 cloves garlic, mashed and chopped
> 2 stalks of celery, chopped

Sauté vegetables until onion is transparent. Add:

> ¼ cup tomato paste
> ½ teaspoon ground cumin
> ¼ teaspoon dried oregano
> ¼ teaspoon black pepper

Add the browned chicken pieces and 1 cup of brown rice. Stir for a few minutes, and then add 1 ½ cups chicken broth. Cover and bring to a boil. Reduce heat and simmer until rice is done and chicken is cooked through, approximately 40 minutes.

Remove from heat and cool slightly. Just before dividing into plastic containers, add 1 cup frozen peas. Put Arroz con Pollo in 6 entrée containers, evenly divided. Add broccoli or other frozen vegetables, put lid on securely, and place in freezer.

Jonni Good

Painted Rooster (Beans and Rice)

This simple dish is extremely easy to prepare, and makes a nice, light change. It is also very inexpensive. This meal often eaten for breakfast in Central America.

Shopping List:

1 can red or black beans
1 onion
Parmesan cheese

Staples:

Brown rice
Cumin

Recipe:

In rice steamer or saucepan put 1 cup of brown rice and 1 ½ cups of water (or according to package directions.) Bring to boil, cover, and simmer until rice is tender, about 40 minutes.

Meanwhile, water-sauté ¼ yellow onion. When the onions are clear and soft, add 1 can drained red or black beans, and ½ teaspoon ground cumin or coriander. Sauté the beans until dry. Stir in rice.

Cool slightly, and divide evenly into 6 plastic containers. Sprinkle 1 tablespoon parmesan cheese over rice and beans, and fill container with frozen vegetable of your choice.

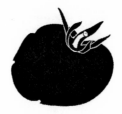

Enchilada Casserole

With corn or hominy

The hominy in this dish makes a very interesting flavor — but yellow corn is nice too. The corn is a grain, of course, so you won't be adding rice.

Shopping list:

1 lb lean ground beef
Onion
Green pepper
1 8 oz can tomato sauce
2 15 oz cans hominy or whole kernel corn
½ cup low-fat cheese
2 pkgs frozen broccoli or other cut vegetables

Recipe:

In large skillet or wok, brown 1 lb lean ground beef, 1 onion, chopped, and one green pepper, chopped. When meet is browned and cooked through, pour off fat, if any. Add 1 cup tomato sauce and 2 cans hominy or whole kernel corn, drained. Mix well. Cover and cook over medium heat for about 5 minutes. Uncover and simmer for 10 to 15 minutes, or until mixture begins to thicken.

Remove from heat and allow to cool slightly. Divide evenly into 6 plastic containers, and top mixture with ½ cup grated low-fat cheese, evenly divided. Add 2 packages of frozen broccoli or other cut vegetables to containers, and place in freezer.

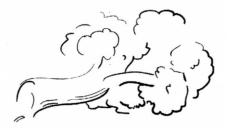

White Bean Soup from Tuscany

With rosemary and parmesan

Shopping List:

2 16 oz cans cooked navy beans
1 yellow onion
1 carrot
Celery
Fresh rosemary (or used dried rosemary)
1 16 oz can low-fat, low-salt chicken or vegetable broth
Parmesan cheese

Staples:

Olive oil
Garlic
Salt and pepper

Recipe:

Put 3 tablespoons of olive oil in a large soup pot and sauté until vegetables are soft, about 10 minutes:

   1 yellow onion, finely chopped
   1 carrot, peeled and finely chopped
   1 celery stalk, finely chopped

Add 2 cloves of garlic, minced, and 1 teaspoon minced fresh rosemary (or use ½ teaspoon dried) and continue to sauté for another 3 minutes.

Drain the water from 2 cans of cooked navy beans. Add the beans and 1 can of low-fat, low-salt chicken broth. Bring to a boil, reduce the heat, and simmer until vegetables are tender, about 15 to 20 minutes. Cool slightly.

Put one-third of the soup in a blender and puree. Return the puree to the soup, and add salt and pepper to taste.

Divide the soup into six individual soup containers, leaving room for expansion. Add ½ cup grated parmesan cheese, equally divided among the containers.

Also prepare six individual containers for frozen vegetables of your choice, using two 16 oz packages. Put the 12 containers in the freezer.

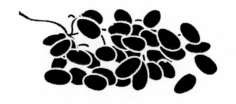

Black Bean Soup

With tomato and sweet onion garnish

This is an old favorite of the Southwest, and for good reason.

Shopping list:

2 cans cooked black beans
1 large yellow onion
1 16 oz can low-salt vegetable broth
2 tomatoes
1 sweet onion
Fresh jalapeno pepper

Staples:

Garlic
Ground cumin
Chili powder

Recipe:

In a large saucepan add 1 tablespoon of olive oil and sauté 1 large yellow onion, minced, for about 10 minutes or until soft. Add 1 to 3 cloves of garlic, minced, 1 teaspoon ground cumin, and 2 teaspoons chili powder. Add 2 cans of cooked black beans, drained, and 1 can of vegetable broth. Bring to a boil and lower the heat. Simmer until flavors are combined, about 20 minutes.

Meanwhile, chop 1 sweet onion and 2 tomatoes, and mince ½ fresh jalapeno pepper, seeds removed.
Remove soup from heat and allow to cool slightly. Divide soup into six individual soup containers. Garnish with chopped tomatoes, onion and pepper.

Also prepare six individual containers for frozen vegetables of your choice, using two 16 oz packages. Put the 12 containers in the freezer.

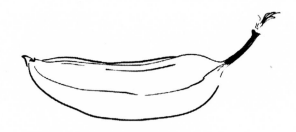

Pasta and Bean Soup

Shopping list:

2 cans cooked white kidney beans
2 strips of bacon (optional)
1 yellow onion
1 15 oz can peeled chopped tomatoes
2 16 oz cans low-salt, low-fat chicken or beef broth
¾ cups (about 3 oz) brown rice pasta
Parmesan cheese

Staples:

Olive oil
Garlic
Sage
Red pepper flakes
Salt and pepper

Recipe:

Mince the bacon, if desired, chop 1 yellow onion and mince 2 cloves of garlic. Sauté in large saucepan with 1 tablespoon olive oil until onions are soft, about 12 minutes. Add 1 can chopped, peeled tomatoes, 1 teaspoon dried sage or 1 tablespoon fresh sage, minced, and pinch of red pepper flakes. Add 2 cans cooked white kidney beans, drained. Add salt and pepper to taste. Simmer over low heat until flavors are combined, about 30 minutes.

Add the pasta to the soup and simmer until the pasta is tender, about 12 to 15 minutes, or according to package directions.

Remove from heat and allow to cool slightly. Divide into six individual soup containers. Garnish with grated Parmesan cheese.

Also prepare six individual containers for frozen vegetables of your choice, using two 16 oz packages. Put the 12 containers in the freezer.

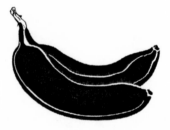

Pasta with Beans and Pesto

With pine nuts or sunflower seeds

Pesto is often served with pine nuts, which can get very spendy. This dish is equally good with sunflower seeds. Or experiment with chopped raw cashews or walnuts, which are fairly inexpensive at Trader Joe's.

Shopping List:

1 can cooked beans (use cranberry, kidney or navy beans or black-eyed peas)
1 ½ cups fresh, firmly packed basil leaves
½ cup grated Romano or Parmesan cheese
1 large yellow onion
1 can low fat, low salt chicken or vegetable stock
1 16 oz package brown rice pasta, any shape
½ cup pine nuts or sunflower seeds

Staples:

Olive oil
Salt and pepper

Recipe:

Rinse the basil leaves, put in blender with ½ cup grated Parmesan cheese and 3 tablespoons of olive oil, and puree.

In a medium saucepan, sauté 1 large yellow onion, chopped, until onion is soft, about 10 minutes. Add 2 to

4 cloves garlic, minced, and sauté for a few minutes more. Add 1 can cooked beans, drained, and 1 can chicken or vegetable stock. Bring to a boil, reduce the heat, and simmer uncovered until the stock is reduced by about one-fourth, about 5 to 10 minutes.

Meanwhile, cook pasta in water according to package directions until tender, about 10 to 15 minutes, depending on the shape. Drain.

Add bean mixture to pasta, and add basil mixture, plus ½ cup pine nuts or sunflower seeds. Add salt and pepper to taste, and combine well.

Divide pasta dish between six entrée containers. Fill remaining space with two packages of frozen broccoli florets. Add lid and place in freezer.

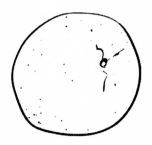

Easy-Does-It Turkey Ragout

Shopping List:

½ lb ground turkey
1/4 oz fresh mint
Small bunch fresh parsley
1 cup dried brown lentils
1 small yellow onion
1 small carrot
1 14 oz plum tomatoes
1 14 oz cans low-salt, low fat chicken stock

Staples:

Garlic
Paprika
Ground cumin
Ground cloves
Cayenne pepper
Salt and pepper

Recipe:

In large saucepan, sauté ½ lb ground turkey in 1 tablespoon olive oil with 3 tablespoons fresh chopped mint, 2 tablespoons chopped fresh parsley, 1 teaspoon paprika, ¾ teaspoon ground cumin, ½ teaspoon ground cloves, ¼ teaspoon cayenne pepper, and ½ teaspoon ground black pepper. When turkey is cooked through, remove from pan and set aside.

Add to the pan 1 small yellow onion, chopped, 1 small carrot, peeled and chopped, and 2 cloves garlic, minced. Sauté until onion is soft, about 10 minutes. Add 1 cup dried brown lentils, 1 14 oz can chopped Roma tomatoes, and 1 can low-fat, low-salt chicken broth, and cooked turkey. Simmer, uncovered, until lentils are tender, about 45 minutes. Season to taste with salt and pepper.

Remove from heat and allow to cool slightly. Divide into six individual soup containers

Also prepare six individual containers for frozen vegetables of your choice, using two 16 oz packages. Put the 12 containers in the freezer.

Barley and White Bean Stew

With Sausage

This dish is so beautiful, with its contrasting green peas and white beans, that you'll want to serve it for company.

Shopping list:

2 cans cooked small white navy beans
3/4 lb pork sausage
2 cans low-fat, low-salt beef broth
18 pearl onions
6 carrots
¼ cup pearl barley
1 lb small red potatoes
1 cup frozen peas

Staples:

Olive oil
Rosemary
Thyme
Bay leaves
Garlic
Salt and pepper

Recipe:

Brown the sausage in a large heavy saucepan over medium-high heat in 1 tablespoon olive oil. Add:

½ teaspoon chopped fresh or dried rosemary
½ teaspoon chopped fresh or dried thyme
2 bay leaves
3 cloves garlic, minced
2 cans low-fat, low salt beef broth
2 cans cooked small white beans, drained
18 pearl onions, peeled, or 2 medium yellow
     onions, cut in large chunks
6 carrots, peeled and cut into 1 ½ inch chunks
1/3 cup pearl barley

Bring to a boil, reduce the heat to low, and cover. Simmer for one 30 minutes.

Cut 1 lb small red potatoes into quarters. Do not peel. Add to stew and continue to simmer for another 30 minutes.

Remove from heat and allow to cool slightly. Add 1 cup frozen peas. Divide evenly in six to eight individual soup containers.

Also prepare six individual containers for frozen vegetables of your choice, using two 16 oz packages. Put the 12 containers in the freezer.

Red Beans and Rice

If you're from the South, you're probably familiar with this favorite dish. Use brown rice instead of the more common white rice, for more flavor and more nutrition.

Shopping list:

2 cans dried pinto or red kidney beans
2 strips of bacon, optional
1 yellow onion
1 red peppers
1 16 oz can tomato sauce

Staples:

Olive oil
Garlic
Hot-pepper sauce (like Tabasco)
Salt and pepper
Brown rice

Recipe:

Place 1 cup brown rice and 1 ½ cup water in covered saucepan or rice steamer and bring to boil. Reduce heat to low and simmer, covered, for about 45 minutes or until tender.

Meanwhile, chop bacon, if desired, and fry in large saucepan until crisp. Pour off excess fat and add 1 yellow onion, chopped, 3 cloves garlic, minced, and 1 red bell pepper, seeded and cut into ¼ inch dice. Sauté until soft, about 10 minutes.

Add 2 cans dried pinto or red kidney beans, drained, and 1 16 oz can of tomato sauce to onions. Add 2 – 3 teaspoons hot-pepper sauce, bacon, and salt and pepper to taste. Simmer until flavors are combined, or until rice is cooked.

When rice and beans are done, remove from heat and allow to cool slightly. Spoon ½ cup rice into six entrée sized containers and top with beans. Add two packages of frozen vegetables to containers, seal and freeze.

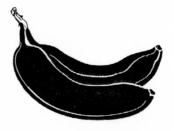

Succotash

With lima beans and sweet corn

Shopping List:

¼ lb bacon, if desired
1 can cooked green lima beans
8 oz package frozen corn
8 oz green beans, cut in 1 inch pieces
1 cup Skim milk

Staples:

Salt
Sugar
Pepper

Recipe:

Chop bacon in small pieces, if desired. Sauté in medium saucepan until browned. Pour off all excess fat. Add canned, cooked lima beans, drained, 1 8 oz package yellow corn, and 1 8 oz package frozen cut green beans. Add ¼ cup skim milk to vegetable mixture, along with a pinch of sugar, and salt and pepper to taste. Bring to simmer over medium-high heat, and stir until most of the liquid is gone. Continue to add milk ¼ cup at a time and cooking until it's almost gone before adding more milk. When all the liquid has been absorbed, remove from heat.

Allow to cool slightly and put in six entrée sized containers. Fill rest of containers with frozen Broccoli florets or asparagus. Seal with lids and freeze.

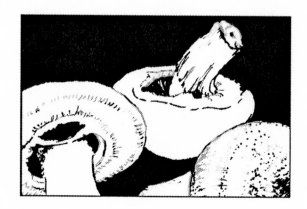

Salads

Every Easy-Does-It Diet lunch and dinner starts with a salad — and there are a number of whole-meal salad recipes included here as well. Salads, with their green leafy vegetables, offer the greatest number of nutrients for the least number of calories. Many of the vegetables that are commonly found in salads, like tomatoes, have been discovered to have micro-nutrients that protect against cancer. All of them help you lose weight.

I know that you may be tempted to skip your salad, especially if you get up a bit late and just want to grab your frozen meal out of the freezer, throw it in your bag, and run out the door. It happens. But try to plan ahead so that you'll have your salad waiting in the 'fridge when you get up in the morning. It makes it easier to have a full, healthy meal for lunch, and the extra effort will help you reach your weight loss goals faster.

Don't stop eating your salads (or your beans!) after you've lost the extra weight. If you keep on eating these delicious meals you'll never have to think 'diet' again!

Use any low-fat, low-sugar dressing that you like. Be sure to read the label.

Green Salads

Green salads can be as simple as a head of loose-leaf lettuce, torn in bite-sized bits, with low-fat salad dressing added. It's definitely green, and it's fast. Many times it's the perfect thing for a busy day, or to accompany more flavorful dishes.

You'll probably also want to get creative, and try every combination. My favorite salad is mixed baby greens, (I buy them in the pre-washed, pre-cut bags), tomatoes, sliced raw mushrooms and a tablespoon each of chopped walnuts and currants. I add a splash of low-fat French dressing, and I'm in heaven. What could be easier?

Here is a list of all the ingredients you can add to your salad, as the whim moves you.

- Apples
- Arugula
- Asparagus
- Avacado
- Bean sprouts
- Beans, green and cooked dried
- Bibb lettuce
- Bok Choy
- Boston, or butterhead lettuce
- Cabbage
- Carrots
- Cheese – low-fat feta, Parmesan, etc.

- Curly endive
- Cilantro
- Corn Salad, or Mache, or lamb's lettuce
- Corn
- Cucumber
- Dandelion leaves
- Dill
- Iceberg lettuce
- Leaf lettuce
- Mesclun (mixed baby greens)
- Mint
- Mustard greens
- Mushrooms
- Nasturtium flowers Oak leaf or red leaf lettuce
- Olives, black or green
- Parsley
- Peas
- Pine nuts
- Potatoes
- Radicchio
- Romaine lettuce
- Red, yellow and green peppers
- Scallions
- Spinach
- Sunflower seeds
- Sweet Onions
- Tomatoes
- Tarragon
- Walnuts

- Watercress
- Whole grain pasta
- Salmon or shrimp

How many of your favorites did I leave out? Some combinations are better than others, so be creative and explore them all.

Whole-Meal Salads

As the name implies, when you take a whole-meal salad to work with you, or serve it at home, it can serve as your entire meal if you add a piece of fruit for desert. That makes it especially easy at lunchtime, because there are fewer containers to carry. This is my favorite way of eating lunch in the summertime, because I can eat my lunch on a park bench near my office and soak up a little bit of sun before going back to my desk.

If the salad doesn't include rice or other grain you can eat a slice of whole-grain bread as well, and have fruit or a fruit smoothie for desert.

The very easiest way to turn an ordinary salad into a whole-meal salad is to add beans, (cooked canned beans or cooked green beans) or frozen peas, or cooked whole-grain pasta, or nuts to your favorite green salad. I often add brown rice pasta and a can of garbanzo beans to my salad, along with lettuce and tomato. Toss with low-fat dressing and you're on your way. If you make your salad the night before, it won't slow you down in the morning.

Another way to make your salad into a whole-meal salad is to add a small can of salmon. In fact, many nutritional experts advise us to eat salmon at least once a week for our heart, and a salmon salad is the easiest way to do it. It's much tastier than the usual tuna salad, too.

Be sure to use the same portion control with your whole-meal salads that you use with your Easy-Does-It frozen meals – no more than 3 oz of meat, if used, and no more than ½ cup of pasta or other grain. You can add any fresh or steamed vegetables, in any quantity. Use a few tablespoons or less of walnuts, raw cashews, or dried fruit like currants or raisins. Nuts and dried fruit are concentrated food, so you need to watch how much you eat. If you have a lot of weight to lose, you might want to leave out the nuts and dried fruits until you've reached your ideal weight.

What About Pasta Salads?

I know you love pasta salads – we all do. But what are they, really? White flour with a few veggies on top, drowned in oil or mayonnaise. They taste great, but – as the ranchers know – the fastest way to get fat is to load up on the grains. Even if the pasta salad were made with whole grain pasta, you'd still only want to have ½ cup per meal – hardly enough to feel full. And you don't need the excess oil.

However, ½ cup of whole grain pasta added to a green salad makes a nice textural change, makes the salad feel more filling, and is a very healthy alternative to pasta salads.

What About Bean Salads?

Although beans are good for you, a bean salad all by itself doesn't make a whole-meal salad, because it leaves out that other great fat-scrubber, green leafy vegetables. By our definition, salads are not just food that's eaten cold – it's a big bowl full of lettuce or other mixed greens, with other stuff thrown in for flavor and nutrition.

Beans can be added to a regular green salad to turn it into a whole-meal salad. About ½ can of any cooked bean, drained, will be a delicious addition to any salad. Garbanzo beans, or chickpeas, have a distinctive texture and are a traditional addition to salads, but just about any bean will work. Experiment with all of them.

If you have a three-bean or Tex-Mex salad recipe that you really love, don't let me discourage you from fixing it. As long as you use reason when adding any oil dressing, you'll have a very flavorful, healthy entrée. Eat it along with a green salad and steamed veggies, and add a piece of whole-grain bread if you're still hungry. Have a piece of fruit for desert. You can also add your favorite three-bean salad directly to your green salad, and toss. Now it's all in one bowl, so it's a whole-meal salad – see? Wasn't that easy?

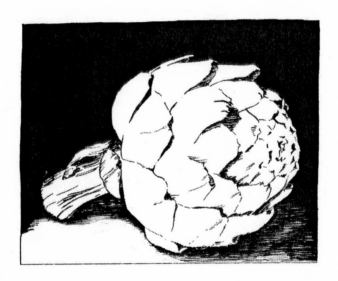

Fruit Smoothies

Fruit smoothies are delicious. They're becoming so popular that many new cookbooks are coming out, complete with beautiful color photographs and lengthy explanations about how healthy smoothies are for you. If you really find you love this way of eating fruit, by all means look through a few of these gorgeous books at the bookstore.

A fruit smoothie, as the term is used in this book, is a mixture of frozen fruit with non-fat milk, yogurt or soymilk, with a tablespoon or less of honey added for sweetener. You'll need a blender to make your smoothie.

You don't actually need a recipe.

To make your smoothie, pour frozen fruit (strawberries, blackberries, blueberries, peaches, mangoes, or whatever you can find) into a blender container up to the one cup line. Pour in non-fat milk or soymilk just to barely cover the fruit. Add one tablespoon or less of honey, into the middle of the container (pouring it down the side doesn't work – it won't blend into your smoothie).

Cover the container and turn it on to the slowest speed. You may need to stop the blender and push the fruit down several times, because the spinning blade creates an air pocket. Always use caution, of course.

When the fruit is well blended, pour it into a cup or glass and enjoy!

To make frozen fruit yogurt, put ¾ cup of non-fat yogurt in the blender container first, add fruit and honey, and blend. Do some experimenting to get the thickness you like — less yogurt or milk will make a thicker shake, more liquid makes it easier to get through a straw.

This is a concentrated food, because of the honey. Research has recently found that honey has some anti-oxidant benefits that can boost the immune system for some people. But use it in moderation, and stick with one smoothie a day until you've reached your ideal weight. If you aren't losing weight on your diet, and you've already given up the whole-grain bread, you may also want to forgo the smoothies and cut back on the other fruit you eat each day until you're back on track.

Or you could go on eating your smoothie, and start an exercise program with plenty of healthy walks and some light weight lifting routines. You'll have faster weight loss results, and you'll get all the health benefits from your fruit.

Once you've tried all the one-fruit smoothies, you can start experimenting with combinations that you think you'll enjoy. One great frozen fruit that you'll never find in the supermarket is bananas. This is a good use for those bananas that are just starting to get too ripe. Put them in a plastic bag and throw them in the freezer, peel and all. When it's time to make your banana-berry shake, take out one frozen banana, use a small knife to cut a strip out of the peel all the way from top to bottom —

you can then just grasp the peel and pull it off. Cut the banana into smaller chunks and throw it in with the berries. I've never tried a banana smoothie, with no other fruit, but it might be good.

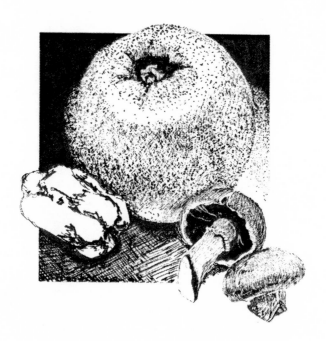

Putting it All Together

I hope that the ideas in this book will get you off to a great start, and that you soon notice a big difference in the way you look feel. Remember to be patient with yourself, give your body time to adjust to the lower sugar and white flour content of your diet, and be happy with slow weight loss over time. It has been proven that a healthy diet filled with nutritious green salads, steamed veggies and beans will give your body the strength it needs to fight of your unwanted pounds.

Also, be aware of your own body and your own needs. If you find you aren't losing any weight, or not enough, then tinker with the program until it works for you. Every body is different. When you're looking for foods to leave out of your diet, always think of the grains first. Go a few weeks without the whole-grain bread, and see if it makes a difference. If not, reduce the amount of fruit you eat, and increase the amount of salads and steamed veggies you eat, if you can. You can also choose to eat more bean dishes than meat dishes, to give yourself another boost in weight loss.

You probably already know that you sometimes to have to fight to stay on your diet, because many well-meaning but ill-informed friends and relatives try to make you happy by giving you fattening treats. How do you stay on track even when people pout because you won't eat their famous chocolate cake, or hang out with them at the local pizza joint?

The easiest thing to do is to gang up on them! Our need to "fit in" and be part of the crowd is so important, and so instinctually ingrained, that the only thing that can keep many of us from giving in to Aunt Betsy's whipped cream and jello "salad" is another understanding soul who's willing to go into battle beside you.

You don't need to start a formal club or anything, but it really helps so solidify some support if you find a diet buddy (or two or three) who are willing to take the process seriously. It really does help if you write up contracts (and this is even true if you're struggling on your own) so that you'll have, in writing, the promises you make to each other. Promise to walk a certain amount every other day, for instance. Promise to share recipes that work well with the Easy-Does-It Diet concept. Promise to call each other before actually eating that candy bar. Promise to have fun with each other, and fun with your diets.

After all – you're on this path because you want to feel better, and look better. What can make you feel better than having friends who understand and support you?

If you can't find anyone in the immediate area, you are invited to come join us at the Weight Loss Success forum. You can find us at http://www.stress-fre-weight-loss.com/forum.htm

I'm always happy to hear from my readers. If you haven't already done so, please sign up for my free weekly How to Think Thin email newsletter, by sending a blank email to **think-thin@aweber.com**

If you would like to send your comments about the book, if you have suggestions for improvements, or perhaps you just want to brag a bit about how much weight you've lost, then please send your email to me at **jonni@howtothinkthin.com**

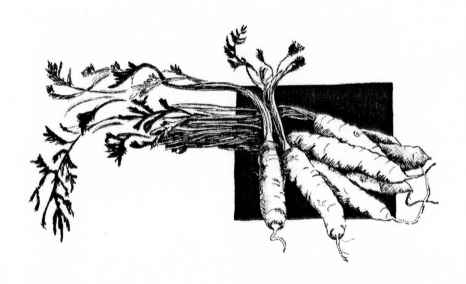